Elective Logbook
for Undergraduate Medical Students

for Block 1 & Block 2
MBBS Batch of _________ Year

As per the latest NMC Guidelines |
Competency Based Medical Education (CBME)
Curriculum under Graduate Medical Education Regulation

Name of the Student: ____

Roll Number/Admission Year: _________________________________

Elective Block 1: ____

Duration of Block 1: ____

Elective Block 2: ____

Duration of Block 2: ____

Elective Logbook

for Undergraduate Medical Students

for **Block 1 & Block 2**
MBBS Batch of _________ Year

As per the latest NMC Guidelines |
Competency Based Medical Education (CBME)
Curriculum under Graduate Medical Education Regulation

Madhulika Peter Samuel

MBBS, MD (Pharmacology), ACME

MEU Coordinator, Medical Education Unit
Associate Professor
Department of Pharmacology
SJP Medical College
Bharatpur

Former Head, Department of Pharmacology
SJP Medical College
Bharatpur, Rajasthan

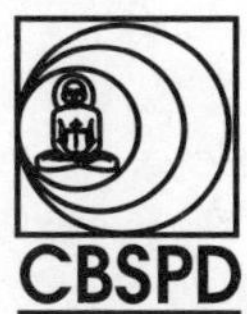

CBS Publishers & Distributors Pvt Ltd

New Delhi • Bengaluru • Chennai • Kochi • Kolkata • Lucknow • Mumbai
Gujarat • Hyderabad • Jharkhand • Nagpur • Patna • Pune • Uttarakhand

Elective Logbook

for Undergraduate Medical Students

for Block 1 & Block 2
MBBS Batch of _________ Year

ISBN: 978-93-49057-03-6

First Edition: 2025

Published by **Satish Kumar Jain** and produced by **Varun Jain** for

CBS Publishers & Distributors Pvt Ltd
4819/XI Prahlad Street, 24 Ansari Road, Daryaganj, New Delhi 110 002, India
Ph: 011-23266838, 23289259

Website: www.cbspd.com
e-mail: delhi@cbspd.com

Corporate Office: 204 FIE, Industrial Area, Patparganj, Delhi 110 092, India
Ph: 011-4934 4934   Fax: 011-4934 4935

e-mail: publishing@cbspd.com;
publicity@cbspd.com

Branches

- **Bengaluru:** Seema House 2975, 17th Cross, KR Road, Banasankari 2nd Stage, Bengaluru 560 070, Karnataka, India
  Ph: +91-80-26771678/79   Fax: +91-80-26771680   e-mail: bangalore@cbspd.com
- **Chennai:** 18/8B, Subbarayan Street, Shenoy Nagar, Chennai 600 030, Tamil Nadu, India
  Ph: +91-44-42032115, 26681266   e-mail: chennai@cbspd.com
- **Kochi:** 42/1325, 1326, Power House Road, Opp KSEB, Power House, Ernakulum 682 018, Kochi, Kerala, India
  Ph: +91-484-4059061-65,67   Fax: +91-484-4059065   e-mail: kochi@cbspd.com
- **Kolkata:** 147, Hind Ceramics Compound, 1st Floor, Nilgunj Road, Belghoria, Kolkata 700 056, West Bengal, India
  Ph: +91-33-25633055/56   e-mail: kolkata@cbspd.com
- **Lucknow:** Basement, Khushnuma Complex, 7 Meerabai Marg (behind Jawahar Bhawan), Lucknow 226 001, UP, India
  Ph: +91-522-4000032   e-mail: tiwari.lucknow@cbspd.com
- **Mumbai:** PWD Shed, Gala no 25/26, Ramchandra Bhatt Marg, Next to JJ Hospital Gate no. 2, Opp. Union Bank of India, Noorbaug, Mumbai 400 009, Maharashtra, India
  Ph: +91-22-66661880/89   e-mail: mumbai@cbspd.com

Representatives

• **Gujarat**	0-9879558667	• **Hyderabad**	0-9885175004	• **Jharkhand**	0-9811541605
• **Nagpur**	0-8692091830	• **Patna**	0-9334159340	• **Pune**	0-9664372571
• **Uttarakhand**	0-9716462459				

Printed at: SRK Graphics, Shahdara, Delhi, India

Preface

By the Lord Jehovah's grace introducing my first elective logbook for MBBS students. As per Competency Based Medical Education (CBME), there is a compulsory posting of elective for each medical undergraduate.

There are many modules in CBME like Foundation Course, AETCOM, etc. but elective is different from others. It is one of the modules which give an opportunity to every student to choose before going in any department.

The logbook is easy to use by students. It is designed in a simplified way for students and faculty. It has an index with proper pages numbers a reflection sheet for every week. It also provides activities table and performance table with daily assessment and feedback by the preceptor. The students will also get feedback at the end of the posting from preceptor. This feedback provides students for improvement in the journey of medical education.

Main idea to conduct electives is to give medical students a small exposure to their future post-graduation branch. This is my small contribution in the medical field. I hope the logbook will help students to achieve bigger in medical life. The student will be experienced in the same department with different prospective during electives.

I want to express my thanks to Dr Suchitra Deolalikar, Professor, Department of Physiology, Smt. BK Shah Medical Institute & Research Centre, Dist. Vadodara, Gujarat, my batchmate in ACME, always encouraging, appreciating and inspiring me. Ma'am always gives me her sincere and very honest comments and suggestions.

I am greatly thankful especially to my father Mr Johnson and mother Mrs Taramani Johnson for their consistent support, love and efforts. I am thankful to my dear husband Reverend Peter Samuel and my cutest son Theophilus Peter Samuel for always helping and encouraging me. Thankful to my dear sister Amita Johnson and brother Mr Sanjeet Johnson for supporting me.

All the best for bright future to my dear medical students.

"I will instruct you and teach you in the way you should go.
I will counsel you and watch over you." Psalm 32:8

Madhulika Peter Samuel
MBBS, MD (Pharmacology), ACME

MEU Coordinator, Medical Education Unit
Associate Professor, Department of Pharmacology
SJP Medical College, Bharatpur
Former Head, Department of Pharmacology
SJP Medical College, Bharatpur, Rajasthan

Student's Detail Information

Name of the Student: ....

Roll No.: ....

MBBS Batch of: ....

Mobile No.: ....

Email ID: ....

Permanent Address: ....

....

Correspondence Address:

....

Parent/Guardian Details

Name of the **Father/Guardian**:

Education:

Occupation:

Mobile No.:

Email ID:

Name of the **Mother**:

Education:

Occupation:

Mobile No.:

Email ID:

Student's Signature

Place and Date

Paste Recent Photo

Word List

Elective

An elective is a learning experience created in the curriculum to provide an opportunity for the learner to explore, discover and experience areas or streams of interest.

Block

Block is a defined time period during which learning experiences are created in a particular specialty, subject or theme.

Logbook

A logbook is a verified record of the progression of the learner documenting the acquisition of the requisite knowledge, skills, attitude and/or competencies.

Activity

This term refers to a predefined task performed by learners that contributes to the achievement of stated objectives or competencies.

Portfolio

Portfolio is a collection of a learner's progression in tasks and competencies. A portfolio is evidence of events documented in the logbook. It includes selected assignments, self-assessment, feedback, work-based and in-training formative assessments, reflections and learnings from planned activity in the curriculum. The maintenance of portfolio is desirable. If a portfolio is not possible to be maintained, an annexure to the logbook can be used for documenting details.

Remedial

Remedial is a planned activity aimed at correcting deficits that prevent a learner from achieving an intended outcome.

Feedback

Feedback is a formal active interaction performed at the completion of an observed activity (or activities) intended to facilitate positive change, growth and improvement of the learner through guided reflection of activity(ies) performed.

General Instructions

1. The logbook is a record of the academic/co-curricular activities of the designated student, who would be responsible for maintaining his/her logbook.

2. The student is responsible for getting the entries in the logbook verified by the faculty in charge regularly.

3. Entries in the logbook will reflect the activities undertaken in the department and have to be scrutinized by the head of the concerned department.

4. The logbook is a record of various activities by the student like:
   - Overall participation and performance
   - Attendance
   - Participation in sessions
   - Record of completion of pre-determined activities
   - Acquisition of selected competencies

As per Competency Based Medical Education (CBME) Guidelines

- It is mandatory for learners (undergraduate) to do an elective.
- This time should not be used to make up for missed clinical postings or other purposes.
- The learner shall do complete Block 1 followed by Block 2 each Block for 15 days.
- The clinical posting shall continue for Block 1 but not for Block 2.

Assessment

- Assessment will be formative.
- Attendance not less than 75% and successful completion of all activities of logbook and its timely submission.
- Assessment includes participation in department activities like attending grand round, presenting seminars, maintain case records, submission of assignments, reflection writing, preparation of abstract for research posters, participation in education programs, etc.

Important Instructions for Electives

1. This **elective module** is designed for medical undergraduates. The students who have **given their final part 1 university examination**. They are supposed to **attend elective module compulsorily.**

2. The electives module will be **starting immediately after completing 3rd Prof part 1 university practical examination.**

3. All students need to **first complete Block 1 for 15 days**.

4. The students will do **Block 2 for 15 days** instantly **after completing Block 1.**

5. The **attendance is compulsorily.**

6. The **students** have to **report in allotted department.**

7. The student should have **75% attendance in Block 1 and 75% attendance in Block 2 separately.**

8. **The Elective Logbook** will be **provided to you.** It should be **maintained by students.** The logbook should be **completed, checked and signed on daily or weekly basis by Preceptor's and HOD.**

9. **The student should have 75% attendance separately in Block 1 and 75% attendance in Block 2 and submission of elective logbook** both are required **for eligibility to appear in final MBBS examination.**

10. **At the end of elective posting, student have to submit Elective Logbook to MEU Coordinator.**

Contents

List of Electives

For MBBS Batch of 2021
Block 1
(Pre-Clinical & Para-Clinical Departments)
Duration
(Roll No: 1–150 & Remaining Students)

Sr. no.	Electives	Preceptor(s)
1.	Anatomy	
2.	Biochemistry	
3.	Physiology	
4.	Microbiology	
5.	Pathology	
6.	Pharmacology	
7.	Community Medicine	

Elective of Block 1–Model

Name of the block	
Name of the elective	
Location of hospital laboratory or research facility	
Name of the internal preceptor(s)	
Name of the external preceptor(s)	
Learning objectives of the elective	
Number of the students that can be accommodated in this elective	
Pre-requisite for the elective	
Learning resources for students	
List of the activities in which the students will participate	
Portfolio entries required	
Logbook entries required	
Assessment	
Any other comments	

Attendance Sheet of the Student

Sr. no.	Date	Morning	Evening	Student's Signature	Preceptor's Signature
1.					
2.					
3.					
4.					
5.					
6.					
7.					
8.					
9.					
10.					
11.					
12.					
13.					
14.					
15.					

Final Attendance Record of the Student

Sr. no.	Blocks	Attendance obtained out of 15 days	Attendance in percentage	Student's Signature	Preceptor's Signature
1.	Block 1				
2.	Block 2				

Important Note

If find any disagreement about attendance, the attendance record of the department records will be considered as final.

Certificate of Block 1

Certificate of Completion

This is to certify that Ms/Mr .... Roll No. .... admitted in the

year .... at ....

has satisfactorily completed/has not completed all requirements of Electives Block 2 in the Elective

.... of .... subject from .... to ....

She/He is/is not eligible to appear for 3rd Prof MBBS Part 2 University Examination.

Signature of the Preceptor

Name and Designation

Countersigned by HOD

Principal Signature

Place and Date

Elective Block 1

Elective Topic: ____

Department: ____

Preceptor's Name: ____

Details of Block 1

Activities Record Table

Sr. no.	Date	Activities	Activities in details
1.			
2.			
3.			
4.			
5.			
6.			
7.			

Activity Performance Status Table

Sr. no.	Name of activity	Attempt at activity **First or Only (F)** **Repeat (R)** **Remedial (Re)**	Rating **Below (B)** expectations **Meets (M)** expectations **Exceeds (E)** expectations	Decision of faculty **Completed (C)** **Repeat (R)** **Remedial (Re)**	Faculty signature and date	Feedback received by student (Yes/No)	Student's Signature
1.							
2.							
3.							
4.							
5.							
6.							
7.							

Reflection of First Week

1. What happened during the first week?

2. What have you learned during the first week?

3. How could that knowledge be helpful in your future?

Faculty Signature with Date

Activities Record Table

Sr. no.	Date	Activities	Activities in details
1.			
2.			
3.			
4.			
5.			
6.			
7.			

Activity Performance Status Table

Sr. no.	Name of activity	Attempt at activity First or Only (F) Repeat (R) Remedial (Re)	Rating Below (B) expectations Meets (M) expectations Exceeds (E) expectations	Decision of faculty Completed (C) Repeat (R) Remedial (Re)	Faculty signature and date	Feedback received by student (Yes/No)	Student's Signature
1.							
2.							
3.							
4.							
5.							
6.							
7.							

Reflection of Second Week

1. What happened during the second week?

2. What have you learned during the second week?

3. How could that knowledge be helpful in your future?

Faculty Signature with Date

Student Feedback

Strengths:

Weakness:

Suggestions for improvement:

Signature of Student
(Feedback received)

Signature of Preceptor/HOD
(Feedback provided)

NOTES

NOTES

NOTES

NOTES

NOTES

Elective Block 2

Elective Topic: ____

Department: ____

Preceptor's Name: ____

List of Electives

For MBBS Batch of 2021
Block 2
(Clinical Departments Including Specialties, Super-Specialties, ICUs, Blood Bank and Casualty)
Duration
(Roll No: 1–150 & Remaining Students)

Sr. no.	Electives	Preceptor(s)
1.	Community Medicine	
2.	Forensic Medicine and Toxicology	
3.	ENT	
4.	General Medicine	
5.	General Surgery	
6.	Obstetrics and Gynaecology	
7.	Paediatrics	
8.	Respiratory Medicine	
9.	Skin and VD	
10.	Psychiatry	
11.	Orthopaedic	
12.	Anaesthesia	
13.	Neurology	
14.	Cardiology	

Elective of Block 2–Model

Name of the block	
Name of the elective	
Location of hospital laboratory or research facility	
Name of the internal preceptor(s)	
Name of the external preceptor(s)	
Learning objectives of the elective	
Number of the students that can be accommodated in this elective	
Pre-requisite for the elective	
Learning resources for students	
List of the activities in which the students will participate	
Portfolio entries required	
Logbook entries required	
Assessment	
Any other comments	

Attendance Sheet of the Student

Sr. no.	Date	Morning	Evening	Student's Signature	Preceptor's Signature
1.					
2.					
3.					
4.					
5.					
6.					
7.					
8.					
9.					
10.					
11.					
12.					
13.					
14.					
15.					

Final Attendance Record of the Student

Sr. no.	Blocks	Attendance obtained out of 15 days	Attendance in percentage	Student's Signature	Preceptor's Signature
1.	Block 1				
2.	Block 2				

Important Note

If find any disagreement about attendance, the attendance record of the department records will be considered as final.

Certificate of Block 2

Certificate of Completion

This is to certify that Ms/Mr .... Roll No. .... admitted in the

year .... at ....

has satisfactorily completed/has not completed all requirements of Electives Block 2 in the Elective

.... of .... subject from .... to ....

She/He is/is not eligible to appear for 3rd Prof MBBS Part 2 University Examination.

Signature of the Preceptor

Name and Designation

Countersigned by HOD

Principal Signature

Place and Date

Details of Block 2

Activities Record Table

Sr. no.	Date	Activities	Activties in details
1.			
2.			
3.			
4.			
5.			
6.			
7.			

Activity Performance Status Table

Sr. no.	Name of activity	Attempt at activity First or Only (F) Repeat (R) Remedial (Re)	Rating Below (B) expectations Meets (M) expectations Exceeds (E) expectations	Decision of faculty Completed (C) Repeat (R) Remedial (Re)	Faculty signature and date	Feedback received by student (Yes/No)	Student's Signature
1.							
2.							
3.							
4.							
5.							
6.							
7.							

Reflection of First Week

1. What happened during the first week?

2. What have you learned during the first week?

3. How could that knowledge be helpful in your future?

Faculty Signature with Date

Activities Record Table

Sr. no.	Date	Activities	Activities in details
1.			
2.			
3.			
4.			
5.			
6.			
7.			

Activity Performance Status Table

Sr. no.	Name of activity	Attempt at activity First or Only (F) Repeat (R) Remedial (Re)	Rating Below (B) expectations Meets (M) expectations Exceeds (E) expectations	Decision of faculty Completed (C) Repeat (R) Remedial (Re)	Faculty signature and date	Feedback received by student (Yes/No)	Student's Signature
1.							
2.							
3.							
4.							
5.							
6.							
7.							

Reflection of Second Week

1. What happened during the second week?

2. What have you learned during the second week?

3. How could that knowledge be helpful in your future?

Faculty Signature with Date

Student Feedback

Strengths:

Weakness:

Suggestions for improvement:

Signature of Student

(Feedback received)

Signature of Preceptor/HOD

(Feedback provided)

NOTES

NOTES

NOTES

NOTES

NOTES

Student Rating

Grade	Rating
A	Excellent
B	Good
C	Average
D	Need Improvement

Summary

Sr. no.	Elective	Date		Attendance percentage	Status (Completed/ Incomplete)	Student's Rating (Grade)	Faculty signature
		from	to				
1.	Block 1						
2.	Block 2						

Signature of HOD